The Anti-HPV Diet:

How I Fought HPV Naturally by Following this Carefully Researched Lifestyle Plan

By Sara Ashley

CONTENTS

MY STORY
STAYING POSITIVE
CHOOSING A DIFFERENT PATH TO HEALTH
ABOUT HPV
PREVENTING HPV
GENITAL WARTS
HOW TO TELL A NEW PARTNER YOU ARE INFECTED
TIPS TO PREVENT INFECTION
CALM DOWN
BECOMING PREGNANT WHILE INFECTED
MY HEALING DIET
RECIPES
MAIN MEAL RECIPES
SIDE DISHES/APPETIZERS
BREAKFAST
PREVENTION RESOURCES
CONCLUSION
ABOUT THE AUTHOR

The Anti HPV Diet:

How I Fought HPV Naturally by Following this Carefully Researched Lifestyle Plan

Copyright © 2016 by Sara Ashley

ISBN: 9781519012036

The content of this publication is not intended to be a substitute for professional medical advice, diagnosis, or treatment. It reflects the opinions of the author. Always seek the advice of your physician or another qualified health care provider with any questions you may have regarding your medical condition. Never disregard professional medical advice or delay in seeking it because of something you have read in this publication.

All Rights Reserved. No part of this publication may be reproduced or utilized in any form or by any means, electronic or mechanical, including photocopying, recording, or by any information storage and retrieval system, without permission in writing from the author.

There is no resale rights included. Anyone caught reselling this book will be prosecuted to the full extent of the law.

The pages within this book have been copyrighted with the U.S. Copyright Service.

MY STORY

When I found out I had been infected with HPV, I experienced a variety of extremely unpleasant emotions. I was angry, embarrassed, confused, and scared. I assume that if you are reading this, you have received a similar diagnosis and are probably feeling some of the same emotions. I hope that by sharing my story with you, you can begin to feel a slight sense of relief by knowing that you are not alone. Although my research suggests that HPV is not completely curable, it can be fought off and lay dormant in your body so that you can live a healthy and symptom-free, life.

I was diagnosed with cervical intraepithelial neoplasia (CIN 3) in April of 2011. I was 22 years old, and had only been sexually active with two people in my entire life (I had thought STD's were for individuals more promiscuous than myself, but I was wrong). I had been getting a yearly pap test since I was 18 years old, and all my results had come back normal until this one. As I understood from my doctor, CIN 3, which is the highest grade of HPV infection before Cervical Cancer, was usually the result of not catching the virus early enough. In my case, I had unfortunately come in contact with a high grade strain and keeping it under control was seemingly difficult for my immune system. My gynecologist told me that my body should be able to fight the virus and assumed it would clear within the next few months. (Apparently, several people who come in contact with the virus are able to fight it without any medical or holistic intervention.)

Because I had just been recently diagnosed, my gynecologist was just going to monitor me every three months to make sure the infected cells did not spread. So, he scheduled me for a colposcopy three months later and advised me of the following to help my body fight the virus:

1. Reduce the stress in my life because stress weakens the immune system.

2. Do not start smoking. (He told me that fighting HPV is basically impossible in the bodies of those who smoke!)

Since I've never smoked in my life, this one was easy because I had no intentions of starting to smoke. Reducing stress didn't sound quite as easy, but I definitely was going to try!

STAYING POSITIVE

Three months went by and I had my follow-up colposcopy to check the infected cells on my cervix. Unfortunately, I still received the same diagnosis of CIN 3. My doctor seemed more concerned this time and seemed to lean towards a more aggressive approach. He said that the best thing for me was to 'freeze the infected cells on my cervix.' This procedure, called a cryosurgery, was supposed to be the answer to recovering my health. After this procedure, I was scheduled another follow-up appointment to see if the cryosurgery had helped.

During the time between the cryosurgery and my next pap, I was in a car accident. I had several broken bones and severe neck injuries. This, obviously, was not optimal for my immune system and it certainly did not help my body fight the virus. Personally, I think this was why it took me such a long time to fight HPV.

A few months later, the next pap test came around, and I STILL was diagnosed with CIN 3. This was not looking good and I was told that I should consider trying a LEEP procedure (The loop electrosurgical excision procedure (LEEP) uses a thin, low-voltage electrified wire loop to cut out abnormal tissue).

CHOOSING A DIFFERENT PATH TO HEALTH

I was tired of going to doctors and always receiving the same negative news so I decided to try a different approach. I am not a doctor and I do not have any medical training. I consider myself an intelligent individual and I understand what is good for my body. While I took much of my doctor's advice, I couldn't bring myself to have the LEEP procedure unless I truly felt it was my last option. I was concerned about the negative effects a LEEP procedure may have for my reproductive system and I did not want to undergo the procedure. In order to feel confident about the (anti) HPV Diet I developed, I did a lot of research on cervical health and natural healing techniques for HPV and cervical cancer. Fortunately, I found some interesting suggestions for improving my immune system to help my body fight HPV. Although I know I will always have the virus and my predisposition for getting cervical cancer is still there, I understand how to keep my mind and body healthy.

I decided to write this book because I know how scared I was during my experience with finding out that I had the virus. I want to share with you my perspective on the virus, how I came to terms with the diagnosis, and how I chose to combat the virus.

Finally, I think one of the most important things I can mention is the fact that when your body is trying to heal itself, it is very important to keep a positive mindset and attitude about your health. I believe medical advice is absolutely important but nothing can substitute your own knowledge of your body. I have made it a life-long mission to care for myself and I take this responsibility seriously. Although I do eat unhealthy foods at times, it is my overall goal to continue to eat a nutritious diet and healing foods as well as get enough rest and exercise to allow my immune system to function normally.

Research suggests HPV clears itself under normal circumstances with a healthy immune system so I looked at different ways to boost my immune system. I will share my findings as well as my lifestyle changes that helped to fight off the HPV, in this book.

ABOUT HPV

Before I learned that I had virus, I had never heard about HPV. One of the reasons I began my blog (cchpv.blogspot.com), was to make more people aware about the prevalence and dangers of HPV so that they can learn about preventing infection. I did a little research on HPV facts and I will share that with you here. I encourage you to do your own research as new information and studies seem to be released regularly on the subject of HPV infection.

Human Papillomavirus (HPV) affects both females and males. It is the most common sexually transmitted infection in the United States. Because it is contagious by skin-to-skin contact, HPV transmission can happen with any kind of genital contact with someone currently infected with HPV—intercourse is not always necessary. Many people who have HPV aren't aware that they are infected because the virus often has no signs or symptoms. Some people get the strain of the virus that creates genital warts but there are several strains of HPV that have no symptoms. This means you can get the virus or pass it on to your partner without even knowing it. If you don't have any signs or symptoms of HPV, the only way to know if you have HPV is by getting an HPV Test. This test can be given to both males and females and is the only way of knowing if you are infected.

It is important to know that HPV can remain dormant in a person's body for years before it is detected. This means you could have the virus and not show any signs or symptoms for years before it causes damage. That is why regular check-ups are mandatory for detection of HPV. Females, especially, should have a yearly pap smear. The pap smear checks the cells on your cervix and alerts your doctor if those cells look abnormal under a microscope. If you have a pap that is abnormal, it doesn't necessarily mean you have HPV. Further testing is required before you finally receive a diagnosis.

(HPV IS NOT THE SAME AS HERPES OR HIV (THE VIRUS THAT CAUSES AIDS). THESE ARE ALL VIRUSES THAT CAN BE PASSED ON DURING SEX, BUT THEY CAUSE DIFFERENT SYMPTOMS AND HEALTH PROBLEMS. HPV IS AN INFECTION AND IT CAN BE FOUGHT IN PEOPLE WHO DON'T SMOKE AND HAVE HEALTHY IMMUNE SYSTEMS.)

In the United States, it is estimated that 80% of sexually active males and females will be infected with HPV at some time in their life. For most people, the virus will clear up on its own within 6-24 months and doesn't cause any additional problems. When HPV doesn't clear up on its own, there can be serious consequences to your health.

There is no way to predict who will or won't clear the virus. However, there are about 6 million new cases of genital HPV in the United States each year. It's estimated that 74% of them will occur in 15- to 24-year-olds.

According to *Journal of Medical Science and Public Health* (1) there are more than 200 types of HPV. The strains of HPV that causes 70% of cervical cancers are HPV types 16 and 18. These strains often produce no physical symptoms and the only way to detect the infection is by getting a pap smear and an HPV test.

HPV can cause normal cells on infected skin to turn abnormal. Most of the time, you cannot see or feel these cell changes. In cases when the body does not fight off HPV, cell abnormalities can eventually cause infertility and/or cervical cancer.

According to EveryDayHealth.com, other cancers that can be caused by HPV are less common than cervical cancer. The following cancers can all be caused by the HPV virus. Each year in the U.S., there are about:

3,700 women who get vulvar cancer

1,000 women who get vaginal cancer

1,000 men who get penile cancer

2,700 women and 1,700 men who get anal cancer

2,300 women and 9,000 men who get head and neck cancers. [Note: although HPV is associated with some of head and neck cancers, most of these cancers are related to smoking and heavy drinking.]

PREVENTING HPV

There are vaccines for both males and females that claim to help prevent individuals from being infected with the most dangerous strains of HPV.

Using a condom may reduce your chances, but it will not completely prevent the spread of HPV.

It seems logical that people who are in a faithful relationship with one partner reduce the risk of becoming infected with HPV. It is also important to note that even people with only one lifetime sex partner can get HPV.

The only sure way to prevent HPV is to avoid all sexual activity.

The Pap Test (for females)

Early detection is important. Even if you are infected with the virus, if it is detected early enough, it is treatable. However, if HPV goes undetected, it may be harder to get rid of and it could lead to cancer.

Your doctor should help you to make sense of your Pap test. Here is a visual that might help you, as well.

The first step is the Pap Test. If this is negative (or normal) then you probably don't run a high risk for HPV infection right now. However, future testing is recommended in order to help prevention. If your pap test is positive and your doctor orders an HPV test, as well, you run a higher risk of cervical cancer. If your pap test and your HPV tests are both positive, you'll need to follow up with your doctor to help to prevent cervical cancer.

HPV TEST	The Pap Test		
	Negative	Inconclusive	Positive
−	Risk of cervical cancer is extremely low. Repeat testing yearly.	Risk of cervical cancer is low. Repeat both tests in 12 months.	Risk of cervial cancer is moderate. Further testing is recommended.
+	Risk of cervical cancer is low. Repeat HPV and Pap test in 6-12 months.	Risk of cervial cancer is moderate. Further testing is recommended.	Risk of cervical cancer is high. Further testing is recommended.

If you have an abnormal (positive) pap test, it's okay! But don't let it go. You can work with your doctor to help boost your immune system, undergo a colposcopy to find out how severe the abnormalities are, and continue to be regularly monitored until your body fights off HPV.

Detecting cervical cancer early with a Pap test gives you a greater chance at a cure. A Pap test can also detect changes in your cervical cells that suggest cancer may develop in the future. Detecting these cells early with a Pap smear is your first step in halting the possible development of cervical cancer.

Coming in contact with HPV is nothing to be ashamed of. You don't have to be promiscuous to come in contact with HPV. The scary part about the virus is that it only takes ONE sexual encounter with an infected person to get it. One source said that HPV is as common as the common cold since 80% of the sexually active community either has it or has had it. However, it is very important to diligently get a pap smear every year in order to catch the virus early enough to treat it. The development of cervical cancer is about 97% preventable when HPV is caught early.

Resources:

(1) Bhardwaj, Subhash, Farooq Ahmed Wani, and Altaf Bandy. "Human papiloma virus testing in the cervix of high-risk women: A hospital-based clinicopathological, colposcopic, and cytogenetic study." *International Journal of Medical Science and Public Health* 4.4 (2015), 538-543. Print. doi:10.5455/ijmsph.2015.13072014110

Other sources:
Centers for Disease Control and Prevention
http://www.cdc.gov/std/hpv/stdfact-hpv.htm
National Cancer Institute
http://www.cancer.gov/cancertopics/factsheet/prevention/HPV-vaccine
The Mayo Clinic http://www.mayoclinic.com/health/pap-smear/MY00090

GENITAL WARTS

HPV is not always a silent infection. Some people are infected with the strain that causes genital warts. Actually, HPV causes all kinds of warts. HPV is to blame for hand warts, foot warts, and the warts that cause cancer. Although there are over 100 noted strains of HPV, here is a small chart that shows a few of the kinds of HPV that cause warts on different parts of the body.

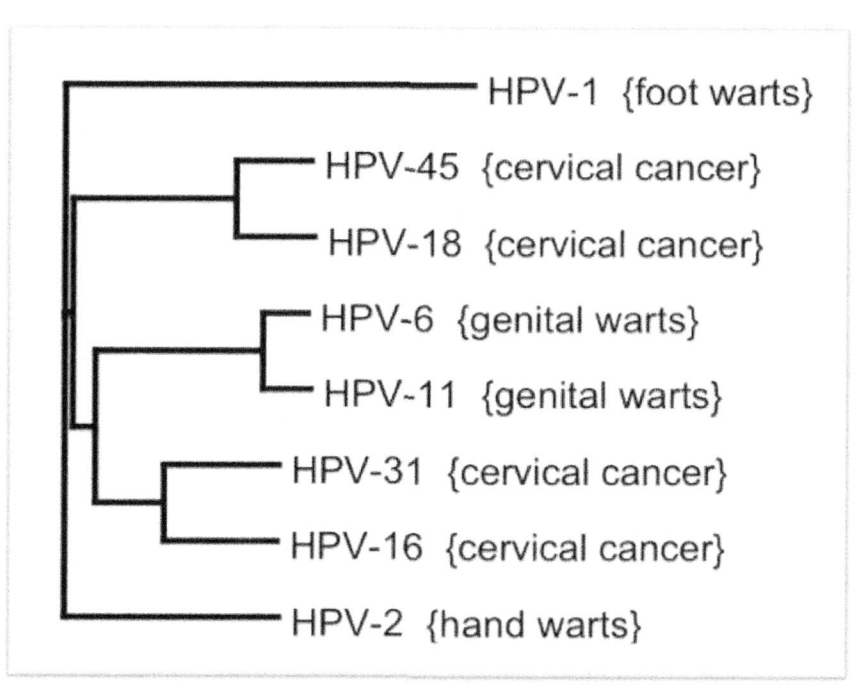

As you can see, HPV infects much more than the genitals and warts appear on many parts of the body. But when you notice a wart in the genital area, it is understandable to be upset.

Genital warts can be removed by a doctor but this doesn't guarantee that they will not appear again. Also, you could have warts internally that are not noticeable. These could be potentially harmful and need to be addressed during a pap test. It is also possible for HPV warts to appear in other parts of the body, wherever skin-to-skin contact has been made. This is why it is extremely important to monitor your body and tell your doctor about any new growths you notice on your skin.

HOW TO TELL A NEW PARTNER YOU ARE INFECTED

I was raised by parents who very rarely discussed sex. I was an only child and I didn't have any siblings to advise me. I was told that I must remain abstinent until marriage and any conversation about sex was extremely uncomfortable in my house. Not to say that my parents did not prepare me well, because they did. But their advice wasn't necessarily as extensive as I wish it had been and I will try to be more open about the conversation of sex with my own children when the time comes.

Because of my upbringing of encouraged abstinence, I was very naïve. I had never even heard of HPV until I learned that I was infected with it. I knew it was a big deal because my doctor was very serious about the news and even spent time on the phone counseling me after telling me the news. I want to spread awareness of this virus and also encourage the conversation about safe sex to be an open one so that there are less people, like me, who find themselves infected because they did not know the risks of sexual intercourse.

When I was infected with HPV, my partner knew he had it and didn't tell me about it until after we had sex. He never actually used the words "HPV" but instead told me he had a wart on his penis he was taking medicine for.

"It's no big deal," he said. "But I just wanted you to know about it." He tells me…the morning AFTER we already had sex.

Needless to say, I was livid. Apparently, he was too afraid to tell me and I was too naïve to ask the right questions. He had the conversation with me the day after the damage had already been done and I scheduled a pap smear a few months after I was infected. That pap was the first of many abnormal smears. I broke up with that asshole far before I received the news of my abnormal pap. I was angry and felt betrayed. I also felt stupid for not directly asking him if he had been checked for HPV. But it's hard to ask the right questions when you don't know the risks. I still feel ashamed that I didn't even know what HPV was until after I was infected.

So many people are infected and don't know about it. But if you do know you are infected, you certainly should tell your partner BEFORE intercourse happens. It is understandable to be embarrassed or ashamed to have to reveal this information in a new relationship, but it is important to reveal this to your partner so that they know risks involved with the HPV infection. Being honest also builds trust in a new relationship.

I probably can't stress enough to you how hurtful it is to be blatantly lied to. I can understand a person not knowing they are infected, but there is no excuse for a person to know about their infection and not let a potential partner know prior to intercourse.

TIPS TO PREVENT INFECTION

-Choose to prolong intercourse until you are clear of the infection. In this case, you should still tell your partner you have HPV but you can explain that it is currently under control. Even if you have had a recent "normal" pap, you can still pass the infection on.

-Always use condoms. Although condoms don't prevent infection, they help to create a barrier and reduce the chances of passing on the virus. You should still tell your partner that you are positive for HPV as there is still a risk for infection.

Words of Wisdom

-In addition to using condoms, always ask your partner if they have ever had an STD. They could innocently think that if they haven't had signs or symptoms that they are STD free. This isn't always the case and you deserve to know.

-Agree to have an STD test before you become sexually active with a new partner. Show each other the results so that neither of you have anything to hide. It is always smart to know what kind of risks you are opening yourself up to and your partner has the right to know your damage, as well.

If you are infected with HPV or any other STD, it is your responsibility to tell any potential partners the truth. If someone isn't willing to listen to your story and try to work out a way to be intimate with you while you are trying to fight off the infection, then they aren't worth your time.

-Plan a dinner to tell your partner before things get intimate. Take the time to be honest and allow him/her to ask any questions they may have about your condition.

-Commit to using condoms at all times in an effort to prevent infection.

-Maintain healthy habits to prevent infection to other places on your body. Remember that HPV is spread through skin-to-skin contact.

CALM DOWN

It is easier said than done…I know. But for your body to completely heal, it is essential to calm down. Learn to balance things in your life. Get your emotions under control because the more stress you feel, the more stress you will create for your body. Stress is horrible for your immune system, so don't allow it to consume you!

Get Your Sleep

The National Sleep Foundation recommends seven to nine hours of sleep per night for optimal health and performance. Most people fall short of this due to a hectic schedule or an inability to fall asleep. During sleep, memories and information are being processed and organized in your brain, so it's essential you get enough of it to achieve clarity.

Reduce Stress

For most of us, stress is the main reason we cannot focus as we want to. Think about stressors in your life and whether you can do anything about them.

-Do not seek out situations you know will be stressful.

-Avoid people who create stress in your life.

-Try to slow down. Think about carpooling or taking public transportation if you feel like you spend your life driving.

-Don't overextend yourself. Know your limits and don't volunteer for too much at work or in your personal life.

For more ideas and recommendations about how to truly calm down and balance your life, check this book out:

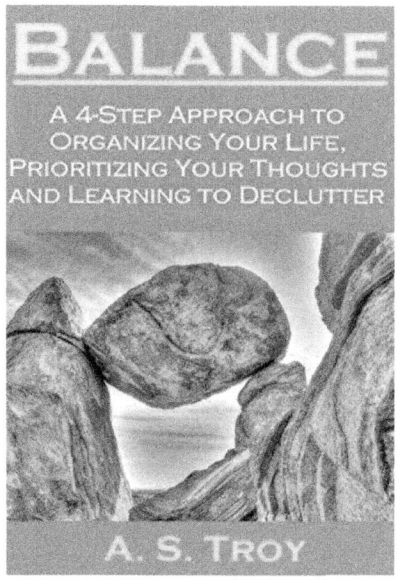

Balance by A.S. Troy hits the nail right on the head and helps focus your mind and body, declutter your world in 4 simple steps, in order to lead a more stress-free existence.

BECOMING PREGNANT WHILE INFECTED

Before I became pregnant, I had a normal pap test which indicated that I wasn't currently infected with HPV. During my pregnancy, I had another pap test came back abnormal. Because of other complications with giving birth, I had to have a cesarean birth. This was relieving to me because since my baby did not pass through the birth canal, he was not infected with HPV.

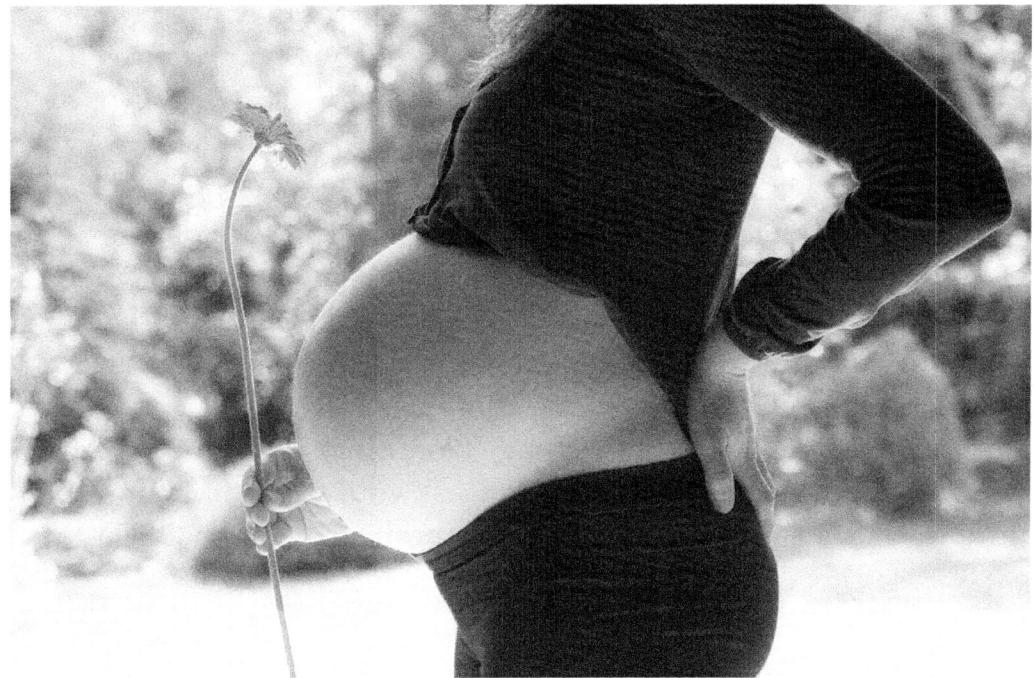

You will need to seek additional medical advice for your specific situation, but there seems to be a very low risk that an infected mother will pass HPV to her child.

Because pregnancy adds additional stress to your body and immune system, it is not uncommon for rapid tissue growth of the virus during pregnancy so it is important that your doctor know you are infected when you become pregnant. Your doctor may need to monitor you more often or perform a colposcopy to make sure HPV is under control.

I was also concerned, before I became pregnant, that the damage from colposcopy and biopsies had somehow weakened my cervix and would make carrying a baby difficult. I'm proud to say that I had no complications during my pregnancy and I have also read several other cases of healthy pregnancies after HPV infection. If you are concerned about the effects HPV may have on your ability to conceive or carry a pregnancy to term, ask your doctor. Most women are able to have healthy babies with the proper care of an OBGYN.

MY HEALING DIET

I researched this diet for myself after I was infected with HPV in an effort to help my immune system fight off the virus. I found that this diet works for me. I'm happy with the supplements and foods I chose and the foods help my immune system stay healthy and ready to keep HPV at bay.

The Supplements

These are the vitamins and supplements I took daily. I took them at the same times every day (except the probiotics, I took those at night on an empty stomach) and I made this part of my daily routine.

Vitamin E (400 IU): 200 to 400 IU of Vitamin E per day has shown to provide a threefold decrease in the rate of invasive cancer. (1)

Vitamin E is also known to be great for your skin. Especially if you are fighting genital warts, vitamin E is essential to skin health. I also use vitamin E as a topical cream. You can even break open a softgel of vitamin E and use it directly on your skin.

Astragalus (470 mg): Increases production of immune-system chemical IL-2, which fights HPV. Activates gene P53. (1)

Astragalus is an herb and its roots are usually used for medicinal purposes. Astragalus is used as an immune boosting supplement for patients with several kinds of cancers.

Vitamin C (1000 mg): Increases immune system function. Vitamin C helps to regrow and repair the tissues in your body. This vitamin is water-soluble. That means that your body doesn't store it. You need to get the vitamin regularly from the foods you eat.

Multi-vitamin: Basically, I found an all around, all-inclusive, multivitamin that would supplement my body. The particular vitamin I took (and still take) is: SOLGAR Prenatal Nutrients. I decided to include this vitamin just to increase immune system function and to ensure I was receiving all nutrients required to fight off the virus. In order to make sure I wasn't getting too much iron, I usually cut a prenatal vitamin in half.

Zinc (30 mg): To improve immune system function.

Aloe Vera Juice: Keeps liver from processing certain toxins into carcinogenic forms. (1)

Aloe Vera is also excellent for skin. It is also an easy-to-grow houseplant. It has amazing healing properties and I use the juice from my aloe plant at home as a topical gel. Just slice a leaf open and rub it on an affected area daily. You can also refrigerate a leaf for later use. I never let this plant go to waste!

I mixed 1/2 cup of liquid aloe vera juice with 1/2 cup distilled water. I drank this before breakfast.

Apple Cider Vinegar: A few laboratory studies have found that vinegar may be able to kill cancer cells or slow their growth. (2)

Garlic: Garlic has antiviral properties and prevents virally infected cells from multiplying, according to James A. Duke, a botanist and author of "The Green Pharmacy Guide to Healthy Foods."

I took garlic two ways:

1. Garlic Tincture: Mix 1/2 Cup of garlic with 1 cup of vodka. Let this mixture sit in a glass jar in a cool, dark place for 2 weeks. After 2 weeks, strain the mixture and throw out the garlic cloves. I took 20 drops with water daily.

2. Chop up one clove of fresh garlic and tape the raw sides to the bottoms of your feet at night time. Take this off in the morning. For those who cannot take garlic internally, or are afraid of "garlic breath," this is a fantastic way for garlic to get into your system without actually ingesting it!

Green Tea: Green tea has many immune system benefits and it deactivates plasmin, a substance that creates pathways for tumors.

Probiotics: To help keep intestinal flora in check, which ultimately improves overall immune system function. (I take probiotics at night on an empty stomach).

Prescription of Herbal Healing by Phyllis A. Balch, CNC. 2002

WebMD, Weight Loss & Diet Plans, Apple Cider Vinegar

The Foods

I changed my diet to be more conducive to helping my immune system fight off the virus. The key is to improve your immune system in order to fight the HPV infection. Here are some of my diet goals and why I chose to do them.

I eliminated all simple sugars. This includes white flour, honey, table sugar, and alcohol. Sugar feeds cancer cells and weakens the immune system.

I reduced my consumption of meat. Meat is very inflammatory and creates an acidic environment in the body. I found that it was much easier to find healthy meals that were vegetarian. I avoided all meat in the attempt to make my body more alkaline. That's why my recipes are vegetarian.

I ate more vegetables! (Veggies make up at least 50% of my entire diet). Mostly raw veggies with nutrients intact, juiced, or lightly steamed.

I ate more raw fruit, and went sparingly on juice as the juice contains lots of sugar without the fiber. I actually mix a class of fruit juice with water so I'm not getting a huge jolt of sugar at one time.

Vegetarian protein is excellent for you- whole grains, legumes, nuts & seeds (brown rice, beans, eggs, almonds & flax).

I Eat Raw Foods / Super Foods as much as possible! (Raw nuts & hempseeds, sprouted grains, goji berries, cocoa, etc.)

Stock up on these tasty snacks (organic and without sugar are preferable): Brown Rice Crackers & Guacamole / Salsa, Fruit and Almond Butter, Seeds and Nuts, Yogurt, Hummus & Veggies, Cereal.

Drinks: Green Tea, Macro Greens, Lemons & Limes for Water, Coconut Water, Rice Milk, Almond Milk.

Condiments: Agave, Olive Oil, Apple Cider Vinegar, Mustard, Stevia, Hot Sauce, Marinara, Salsa, Butter.

Additions: Curry, Pesto, Seasonings, Cilantro, Black Olives, Artichoke Hearts, Coconut Milk, Cinnamon.

Some things about food that I didn't know...

-Yes, you can get plenty of calcium without eating dairy!

-Yes, you can get plenty of protein without eating animal meat! (And actually, you don't need nearly as much protein as you think.)

-Drinking more water actually curbs your appetite!

I think it is important to note that this diet must be a lifestyle change in and of itself. Once I chose to eat these foods I never stopped eating them. Today, I am lenient, at times, and do not adhere to a strict diet since I feel that I have built my immune to a level where it can keep HPV at bay. In order to be a truly healthy person with an immune system able to fight viruses, it is important to eat a healthy diet as outlined and do your best to eat well balanced and nutritious meals. In other words, instead of thinking of this as a temporary diet, you should try to continue to incorporate some of these healthy ideas into your life from here on out. I followed this diet strictly for 6 months. After 6 months, I started to eat more meats and dairy.

LIFESTYLE CHANGES

Healing my body meant changing some things in my routine. I looked at habits that may not be beneficial to my immune system. I decided to get more sleep and become more positive in my thoughts. I never smoked, but I know people with HPV who do. Smoking is the worst thing you can do while you have an HPV infection and you should stop indefinitely.

Quit Smoking

The first question I was asked upon my diagnosis was if I smoked. I don't smoke, but I was curious why this seemed to be a huge deal. I know smoking isn't good for you but I decided to do a little research to find out exactly why it was absolutely imperative to not smoke if you are infected with HPV.

According to "Clearance of Oncogenic Humanpapilloma virus (HPV) Infection: effect of smoking," smoking is associated with a reduced probability of clearing the HPV infection. Aside from reducing the immune system response, the carcinogens of the cigarette smoke seemed to help feed HPV and cancers.

Source: (http://link.springer.com/article/10.1023/A:1020668232219#page-1)

Besides knowing smoking is not a healthy habit, it is very important to quit smoking if you are infected with HPV. Since smoking weakens the immune system, it makes fighting the virus nearly impossible.

Get Enough Sleep

We have always heard that getting enough sleep is important to the overall health of your body. I read an article that explained the concept very well. "Sleep and the Immune System" by Daniel P. Cardinali, and Ana I. Esquifino explain how The 24 hour sleep/wake rhythm correlates with specific circadian patterns of immune responses. During a study, the authors found clinical evidence that the balancing function of sleep is important to immune system response. This is indicated by the findings of an increased allergic skin reaction after sleep deprivation in patients with atopic dermatitis. Because the sleep rhythms were altered for only half the patients in the study, the patients who did not get sufficient sleep were unable to fight off dermatitis as well as others who had an uninterrupted session of sleep. I'd imagine that to be the same with those of us fighting off HPV. Unlike dermatitis, HPV is not something able to be seen without a microscope so the effects of sleep deprivation is less obvious but certainly it is still an important factor to consider when thinking about boosting your immune system response.

Source: (http://www.ingentaconnect.com/content/ben/cir/2012/00000008/00000001/art00009)

Exercise

I enjoy hiking and try to get my exercise regularly. Not only is exercising wonderful for your body and helps to keep you in shape, has it also helps to increase the power of your immune system. Even an extra 5 minute walk a day helps reduce stress. Try these simple tricks for getting a little extra exercise into your day:

- Park as far as you can from the door of the grocery store. This makes you walk further and helps get some extra exercise into your day.
- Take the stairs instead of the elevator.
- Practice simple stretches or light cardio while watching evening television.
- Stand up more. Even if you have a desk job, try typing in the standing position for a while.

While going to a gym may be optimal for some people to get a daily work out, most people don't find the time to do this each day. Doing simple things and changing habits is a good start and you will feel healthier while you're making this lifestyle change!

Becoming Positive

Your mindset can go a long way as far as fighting off a virus is concerned. I found it very important to shift my mindset from feeling so many negative emotions to harnessing gratitude in my everyday life. I began volunteering and practicing yoga as a way to find positivity in my life and to feel more positive about my situation.

Practicing gratitude daily is a great way to promote positivity in your daily routine. Some people enjoy yoga, which is as much an exercise of the mind as it is physical.

Keeping a journal also helps to express negative emotions in a productive way-allowing you to feel negative emotions and get it out on paper is a therapeutic practice for many people.

Take time for yourself every day. Just like it is important to take time to prepare healthy foods to eat, taking time to think and relax is important for you, too. Resting is essential to your immune system and your overall health.

Any way that you choose to be positive and happy, remember that this is a necessary part of healing your body holistically inside and out.

RECIPES

The hardest thing for me was figuring out what to eat. Basically everything you buy at a store has sugar, honey, or high fructose corn syrup...So really, what do you eat?! I had to make my own food from my own recipes. Because of my busy lifestyle, I found that it was much easier to make some of this food in bulk and just save it for later by freezing it.

Some things you may want to pick up:

Oat flour (or just throw rolled oats in the blender until they are the consistency of flour)

Almond flour (or put almonds in the blender until they look like flour)

Stevia (this is an herb that serves as a natural sweetener)

MAIN MEAL RECIPES

Black Bean Veggie Burger

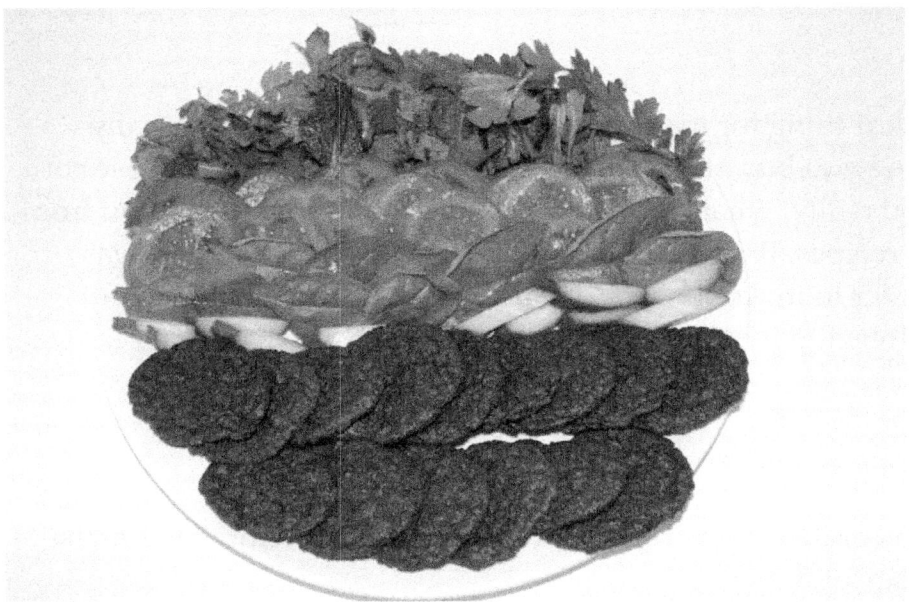

(Makes about 6 burgers)

Ingredients:

½ Cup cooked brown rice

½ Cup cooked black beans

½ Cup finely chopped/pureed vegetables of your choice

Salt and Pepper to taste

Garlic Powder to taste

Instructions:

To make one burger mash together cooked brown rice and cooked black beans. Add finely chopped or pureed veggies of your choice and add a pinch of salt and pepper and any other spices to taste. Shape into burger patties. Heat olive oil in a pan and add the patties. Cook until crispy. Add sauce of choice (I love Guacamole...) add chopped tomatoes and lettuce. Sandwich between a whole wheat bun or tortilla.

Pureed Pumpkin Soup

Ingredients:

4 Cups pumpkin puree

2 cloves of raw garlic

Cinnamon and salt and pepper to taste

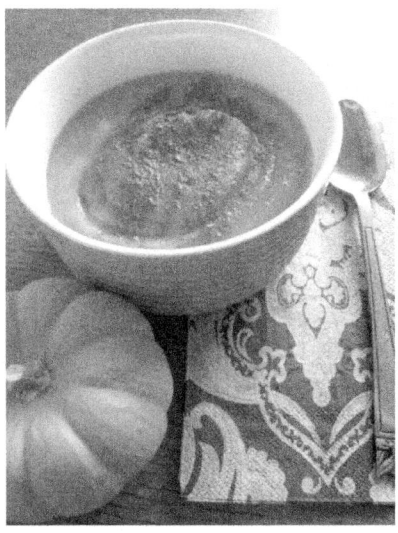

Instructions:

*Since I baked a pumpkin and pureed it myself, I did not need to add any water to my soup. However, if you are using canned pumpkin and it is very thick, you may need to add some water.

In a deep pot mix pumpkin puree, garlic, and spices together with a hand blender. Serve warm.

Potato Soup

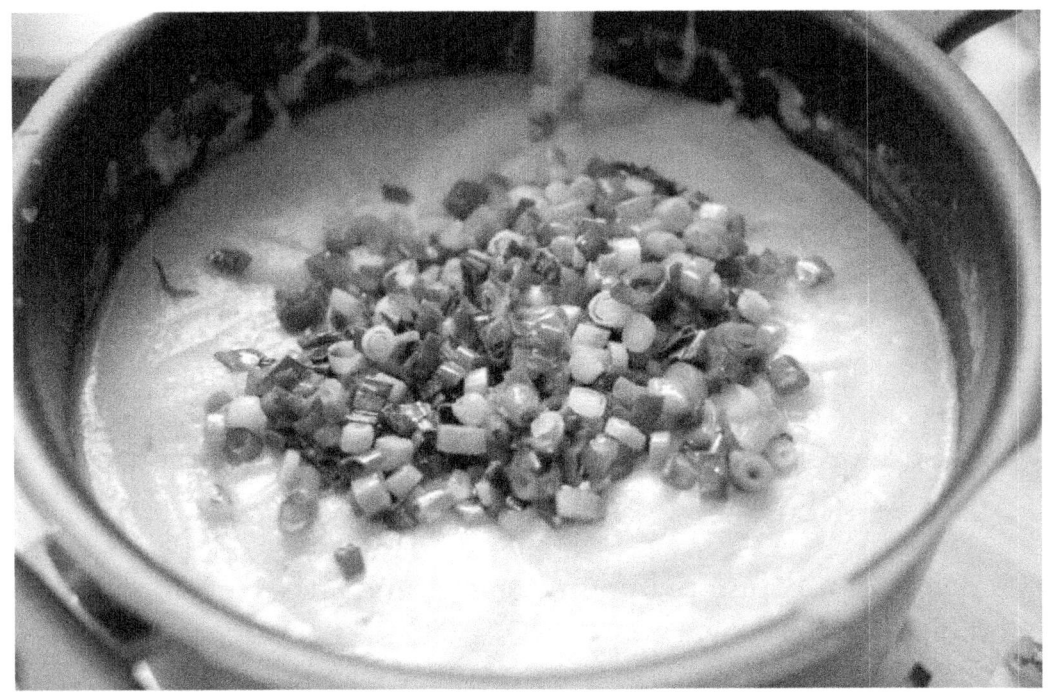

Ingredients:

½ onion, diced

3 cloves garlic, minced

1 head cauliflower, cut into 1 - 2 inch florets

2 pounds Russet potatoes, unpeeled and cut into 1 inch cubes

6 cups water

1 cup almond milk

1½ teaspoons salt (if using store bought broth, taste test after only 1 teaspoon)

Pepper, to taste

Recommended toppings: sliced green onions and chopped tomatoes

Instructions:

I put all these ingredients (except almond milk) in the slow cooker and cook on low for 6-8 hours. Add almond milk when ready to serve. Then I use a hand mixer to puree the larger chunks. If you don't want to use the slow cooker, bring water to a boil and simmer all ingredients in a pot on the stove for about 45 minutes and then puree it to smooth out the chunks.

Vegetable Soup

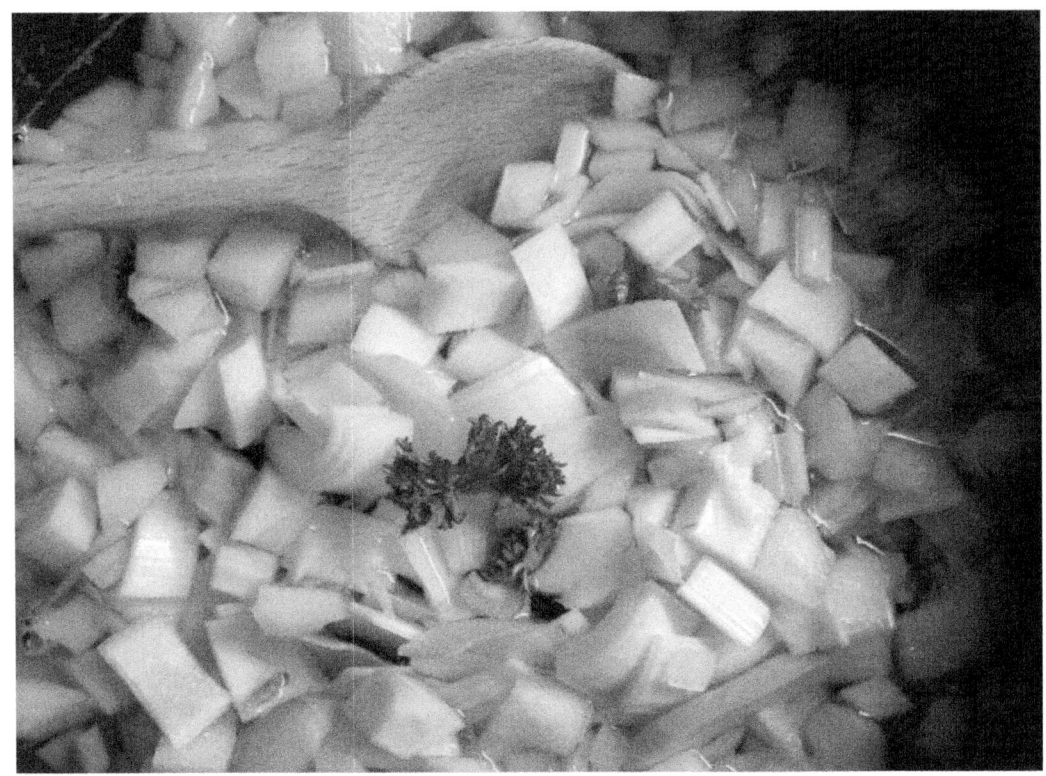

Ingredients:

1 red onion, chopped

2 large carrots, chopped

2 sticks celery, chopped

1 medium sweet potato, chopped

2 garlic cloves, minced

1 can (28 oz.) diced tomatoes

4 cups vegetable stock or water

2 tsp. fresh sage leaves, chopped

A few cabbage leaves, shredded

Sea salt and freshly ground black pepper to taste

Instructions:

I put all these ingredients in the slow cooker and cook on low for 6-8 hours. Then I use a hand mixer to puree the vegetable chunks. If you don't want to use the slow cooker, bring water to a boil and simmer all ingredients in a pot on the stove for about 45 minutes and then puree it to smooth out the veggie chunks.

Spaghetti Squash and Marinara

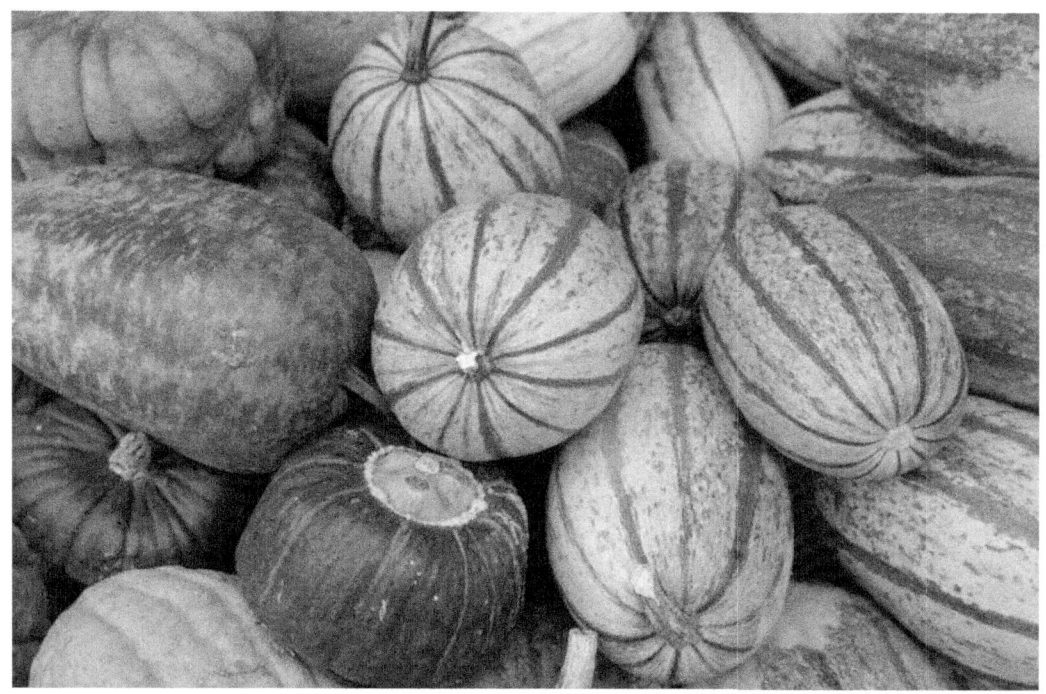

Ingredients:

2 Ounces Black Olives

4 Cloves Garlic

1 Bunch Fresh Oregano

1 Yellow Onion

1 Spaghetti Squash

1 15-Ounce Can Diced Tomatoes

3 tablespoons olive oil

Instructions:

Preheat the oven to 450°F. Wash and dry the fresh produce. Using a sharp, sturdy knife, carefully halve the squash lengthwise. Cut off and discard the mushroom stems; medium dice the caps. Peel and mince the garlic. Peel and small dice the onion. Pick the oregano leaves off the stems; discard the stems and roughly chop the leaves. <u>Using the flat side of your knife, smash the olives; remove and discard the pits, then roughly chop.</u> Place the squash halves on a high-sided sheet pan (or baking dish). Drizzle the cut sides with olive oil and season with salt and pepper. Arrange the squash halves cut sides down and drizzle the skin sides with olive oil. Fill the pan with ¼ inch of water. Roast 28 to 32 minutes, or until the cut sides are tender when pierced with a knife. Remove from the oven and set aside to cool. While the squash roasts, in a medium pot, heat 2 teaspoons of olive oil on medium until hot. Add the onion, garlic, and mushrooms; season with salt and pepper. Cook, stirring occasionally, 6 to 8 minutes, or until softened. Add the diced tomatoes; season with salt and pepper. Cook, stirring occasionally, 10 to 12 minutes, or until slightly thickened. Turn off the heat and stir in half of the oregano. Set aside in a warm place. Once the roasted squash is cool enough to handle, using a large spoon, scrape out and discard the seeds and pulp. Gently scoop the flesh out of the skin in one large piece. Transfer to a large bowl. Using your hands, gently break the flesh into long, thin strands. (The result should resemble cooked spaghetti.) In a large pan, heat some olive oil and 3 tablespoons on medium heat. Add the squash strands; season with salt and pepper. Cook, stirring occasionally, 2 to 4 minutes, or until the water has evaporated. Remove from heat.

Cholay

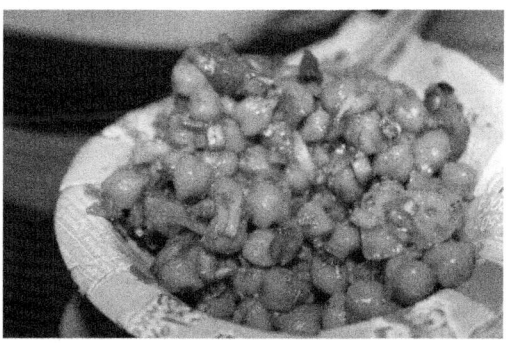

Ingredients:

2 tablespoons olive or grape seed oil

3/4 cup yellow onion, diced

1-2 cups tomatoes, roughly chopped and drained of any water or juices

1 tablespoon minced garlic

1 jalapeño pepper, seeds and stem removed

1/4 teaspoon sea salt

1/8 teaspoon ground black pepper

1/4 teaspoon chili powder (or more for added heat)

1/2 teaspoon curry powder

1/4 teaspoon ground turmeric

1 teaspoon ground cumin

1/2 teaspoon ginger powder

1/2 teaspoon coriander seeds, crushed

2 bay leaves

3 cups cooked chickpeas (garbanzo beans)

Freshly chopped cilantro

Directions:

Heat oil in a medium-sized, deep bottom sauce pan. Add the onions and sauté until translucent. Add tomatoes and garlic. Dice the jalapeño then add the dried spices. Cook down for 1-2 minutes then add the chickpeas. Taste for spice and adjust, if necessary. Reduce heat to low-medium and cook, uncovered for 10-12 minutes. Sprinkle fresh cilantro on top just before serving.

SIDE DISHES/APPETIZERS

Black Bean and Corn Salad

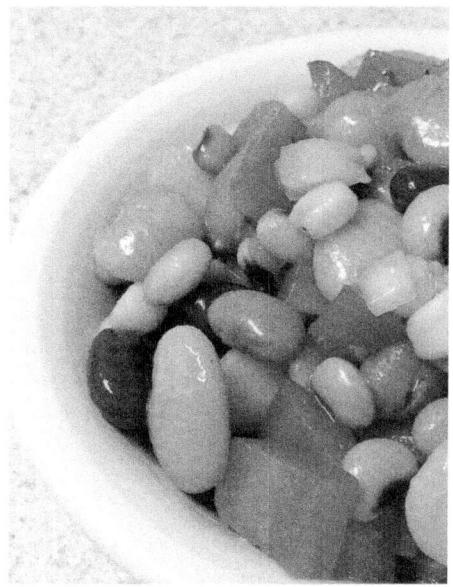

Ingredients:

2 cups cooked black beans, rinsed and drained
2 cups frozen corn kernels
1 small red bell pepper, seeded and chopped
1 red onion, chopped
1 1/2 teaspoons ground cumin
2 teaspoons hot sauce

1 lime, juiced and seeded
2 tablespoons olive oil
Salt and pepper to taste

Directions:

Combine all ingredients in a bowl. Let stand at least 15 minutes for corn to fully defrost and flavors to combine, then toss and serve.

Carrot Fries

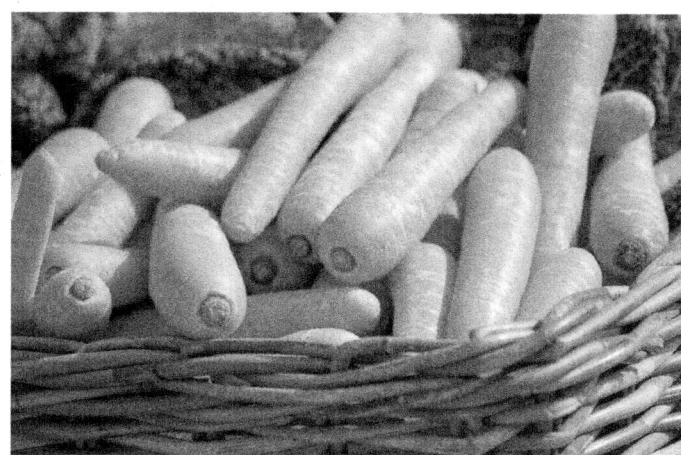

Ingredients:

2 lbs carrots

1 tablespoon olive oil

salt and pepper to taste

Directions:

Preheat oven to 425 degrees. Peel and slice carrots into french fry shaped pieces. Toss carrots with olive oil, salt and pepper. Arrange carrots in a single layer on baking sheet. Bake for 15 minutes then flip each carrot fry. Continue to bake until fully cooked and slightly crispy, about an additional 15 minutes.

Vegetarian Cabbage Rolls

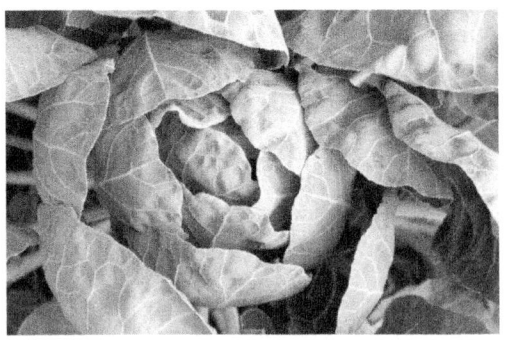

Ingredients:

1 cup diced zucchini

¾ cup chopped green pepper

¾ cup chopped sweet red pepper

¾ cup water

½ cup brown rice (cooked)

1 teaspoon dried basil

½ teaspoon dried marjoram

½ teaspoon dried thyme

¼ teaspoon pepper

1 large head cabbage

2 teaspoons lemon juice

1 can (8 ounces) tomato sauce

1/8 teaspoon hot sauce

Directions:

In a large saucepan, combine the first 10 ingredients. Bring to a boil over medium heat. Reduce heat; cover and simmer for 5 minutes. Remove from the heat; let stand for 5 minutes.

Meanwhile, cook cabbage in boiling water just until leaves fall off head. Set aside eight large leaves for rolls (refrigerate remaining cabbage for another use). Cut out the thick vein from each leaf, making a V-shape cut. Overlap cut ends before filling. Place a heaping 1/3 cupful on each cabbage leaf; fold in sides. Starting at an unfolded edge, roll the cabbage to completely enclose filling. Combine tomato sauce and hot sauce; pour 1/3 cup into a 2-qt. baking dish. Place cabbage rolls in dish; spoon remaining sauce over top. Cover and bake at 400° for 15 minutes or until heated through.

BREAKFAST

Banana Pancakes

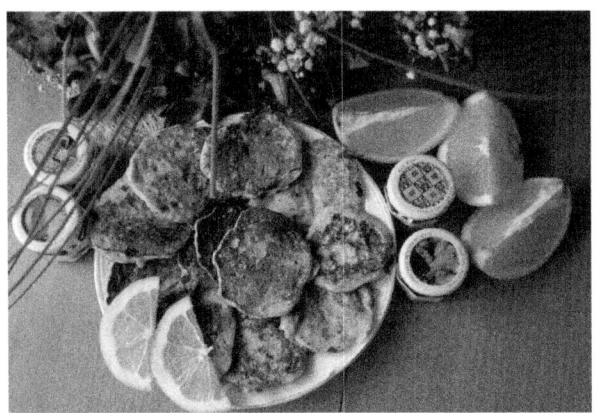

1 cup oat flour

1 tablespoon white sugar

2 tsp baking powder

1/4 tsp salt

1 egg beaten

1 cup almond milk

2 TBSP Olive Oil

2 ripe bananas mashed

Combine flour, white sugar, baking powder and salt. In a separate bowl, mix together egg, milk, vegetable oil and bananas.

Stir flour mixture into banana mixture; batter will be slightly lumpy.

Heat a lightly oiled griddle or frying pan over medium high heat. Pour or scoop the batter onto the griddle, using approximately 1/4 cup for each pancake. Cook until pancakes are golden brown on both sides; serve hot.

Oatmeal

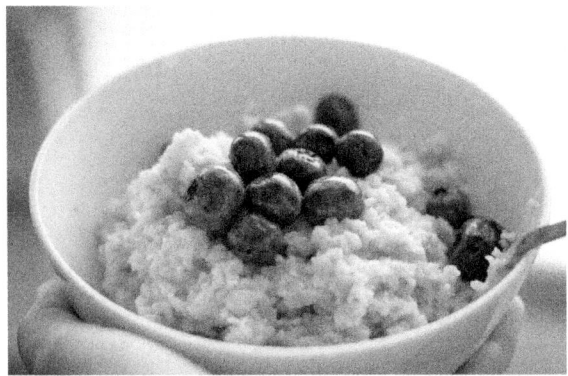

1 Cup rolled oats

1 ½ Cup water

 Suggested toppings:

Raisins

Chopped fruit

Agave or stevia

Mix oats and water together and boil until mixture is creamy and the water is combined completely with oats. Top with favorite toppings.

Delicious Omelet

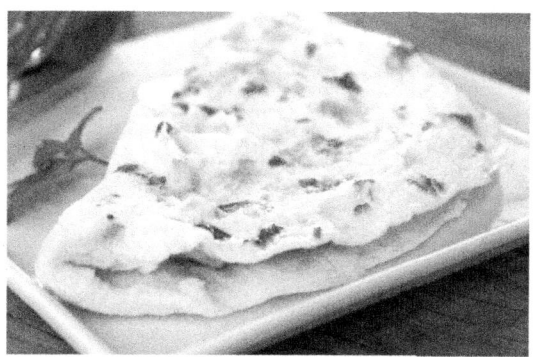

Ingredients:

2 Eggs

Salt & Pepper

Seasonings of your choice

Directions:

Scramble together 2 eggs, all purpose seasoning & a pinch of salt and pepper. Cook diced peppers and onions in a small skillet with butter. Add scramble and turn down heat to medium. Lift edges of omelet to allow runny top to drain under and cook. Once top is not runny, flip! (This takes practice). Immediately turn off heat and let continue to cook for only about 30 seconds. Flip over in half and enjoy! I used Almond or Peanut Butter spread).

Applesauce Pumpkin Bread

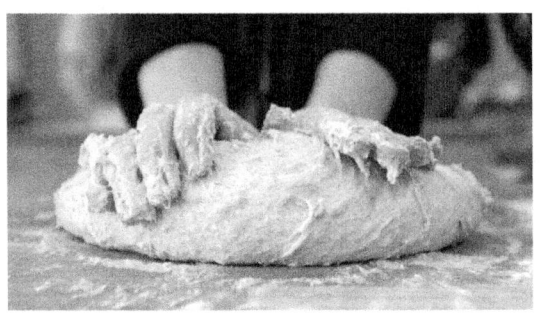

INGREDIENTS:

1 cup whole wheat flour

1 cup oat flour

1 tablespoon baking powder

1 tablespoon pumpkin pie spice (no sugar added)

2 eggs

1/3 cup agave

1 cup apple sauce (no sugar added)

1/4 cup unsweetened almond milk

1 (15 ounce) can pumpkin (NOT pumpkin pie filling)

Directions:

In a large bowl, whisk together the flour, baking powder and pumpkin pie spice. In a separate bowl, combine the remaining ingredients and whisk to combine. Combine the liquid into the flour and stir until smooth. Spoon mixture into greased mini muffin tins. Bake at 350 degrees F. for 40-50 minutes.

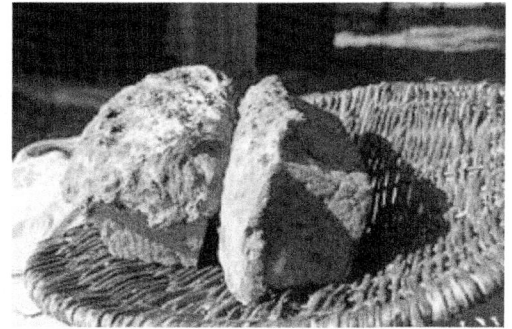

PREVENTION RESOURCES

HPV Information and Resources

Centers for Disease Control and
Prevention: http://www.cdc.gov/hpv/resources.html
Gardasil Vaccination
Information: http://www.immunize.org/vis/vis-hpv-gardasil.pdf
Cervarix Vaccination
Information: http://www.immunize.org/vis/vis-hpv-cervarix.pdf
Inspire: http://www.inspire.com/groups/national-cervical-cancer-coalition/

FREE Pap Smear Resources:

Local county health departments and women's clinics offer free and low cost Pap smears. For the uninsured, cost of the test is usually based on income level.

The National Breast and Cervical Cancer Early Detection is a federally funded program that assists uninsured and impoverished women in getting regular Pap smears. The program is available to eligible women ages 18 to 64.

Here is another link for information on Pap Tests:
http://www.cdc.gov/cancer/nbccedp/screenings.htm

CONCLUSION

I hope this book helps you to create a plan of action for yourself. HPV is a nasty little virus but it, alone, won't kill you. As long as you stay diligent with your health, cervical cancer should be preventable.

I encourage you to seek professional medical advice and follow the directions of your medical practitioner. I also encourage you to follow your heart because no one knows your body better than you.

Take health into your own hands by taking care of yourself. This body is the only one you'll ever have and it is important to treat it well.

I understand the frustration you may feel when you continue to get bad news of abnormal pap tests. Even after your body clears the virus, you may have an abnormal test later in life. The important thing is to never lose hope.

There may be no cure for HPV but there are so many resources out there for you to use. There are many resoures for low-income individuals and the uninsured. Make sure you take care of your health and take advantage of these resources.

To continue the conversation about fighting HPV, let's stay connected!

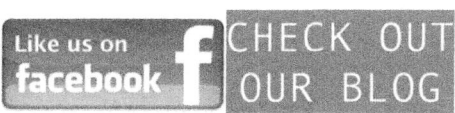

All the best!

ABOUT THE AUTHOR

Sara Ashley began researching the HPV diet when she was diagnosed in 2011 and finally became cleared of the infection in 2014, in time to deliver a healthy baby boy free of infection from HPV. Sara created the blog: cchpv.blogspot.com in an effort to spread awareness and prevention of Cervical Cancer and HPV.

Printed in Great Britain
by Amazon